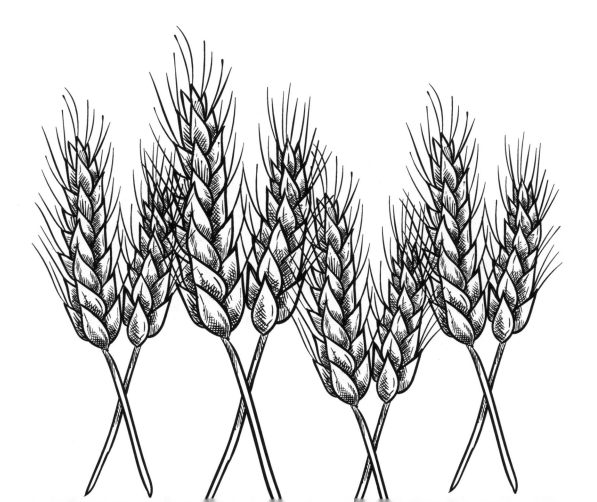

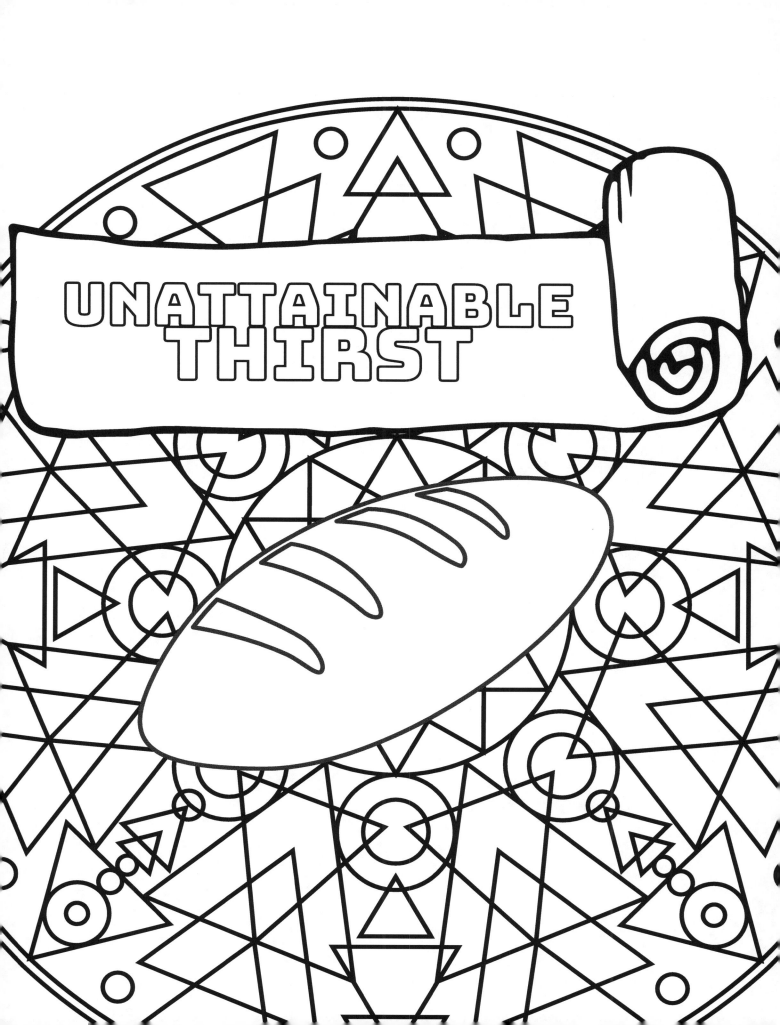

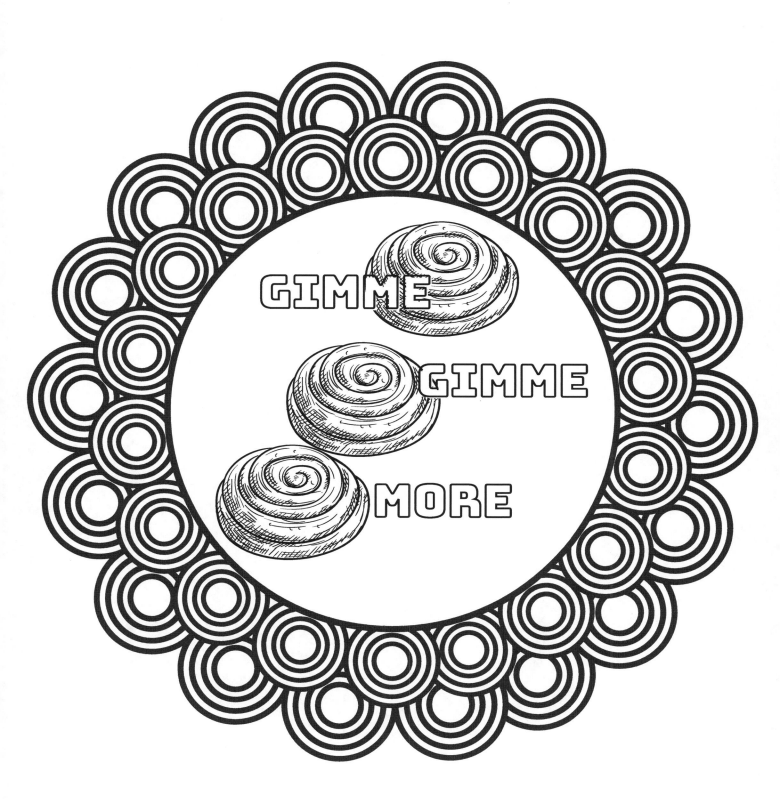

celiac
disease

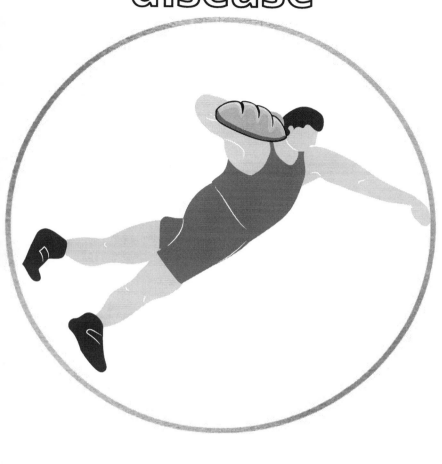

my life

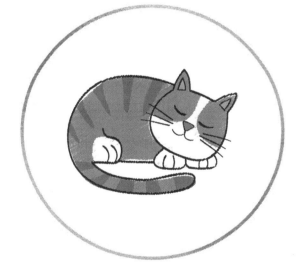

place for your
TEARS

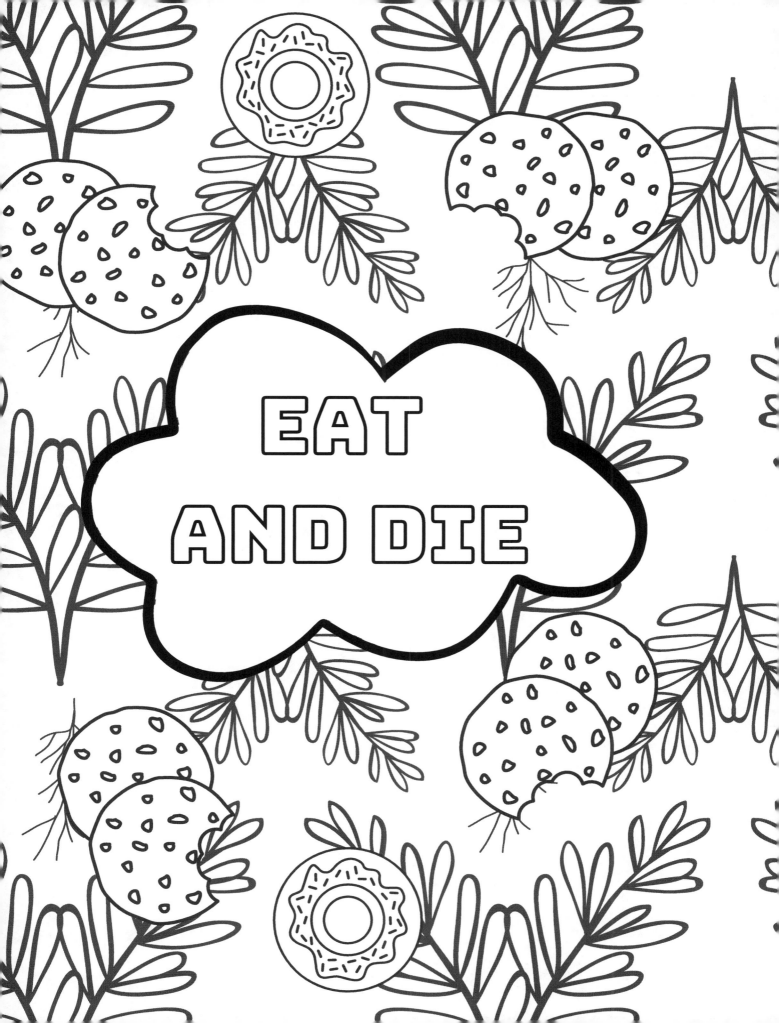

They say:
create healthy
habits,
not restrictions

As if that was easy

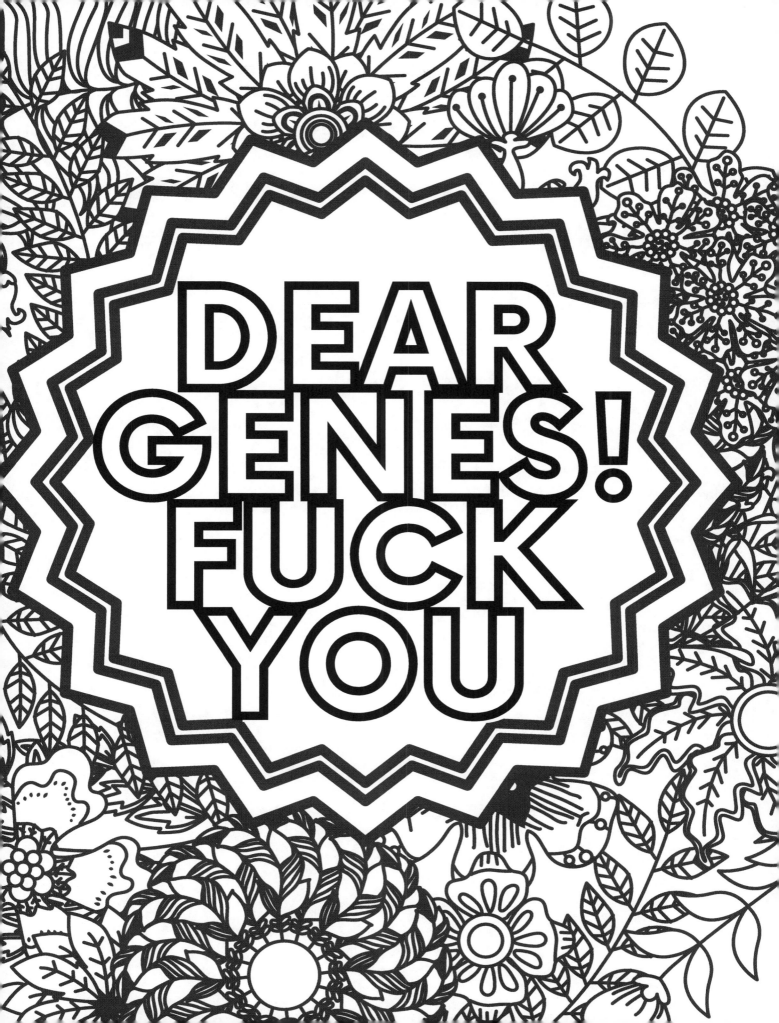

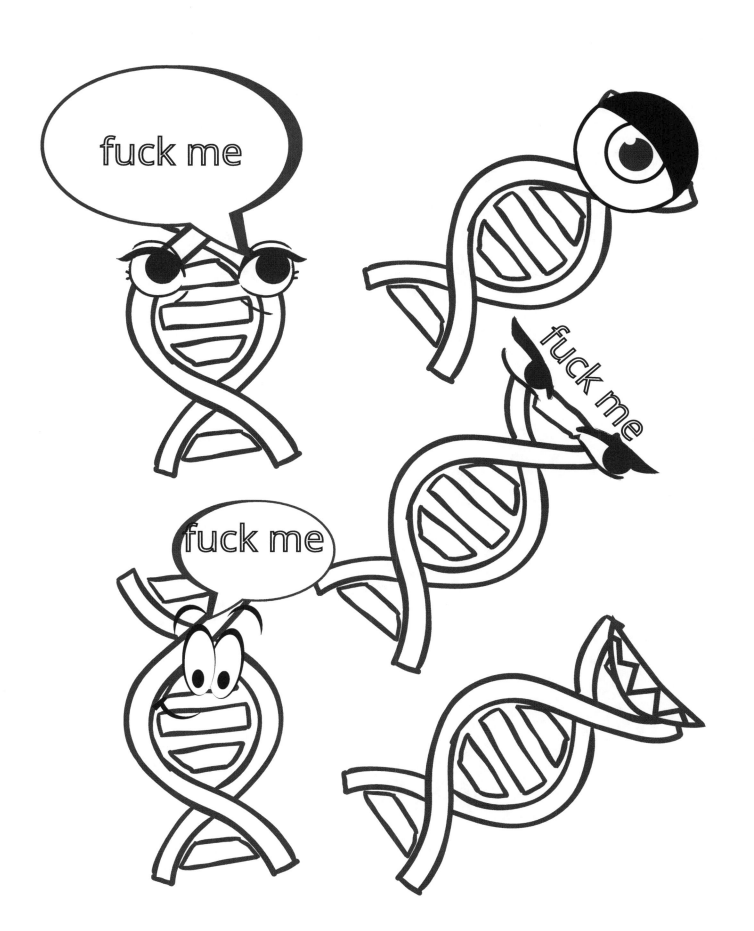

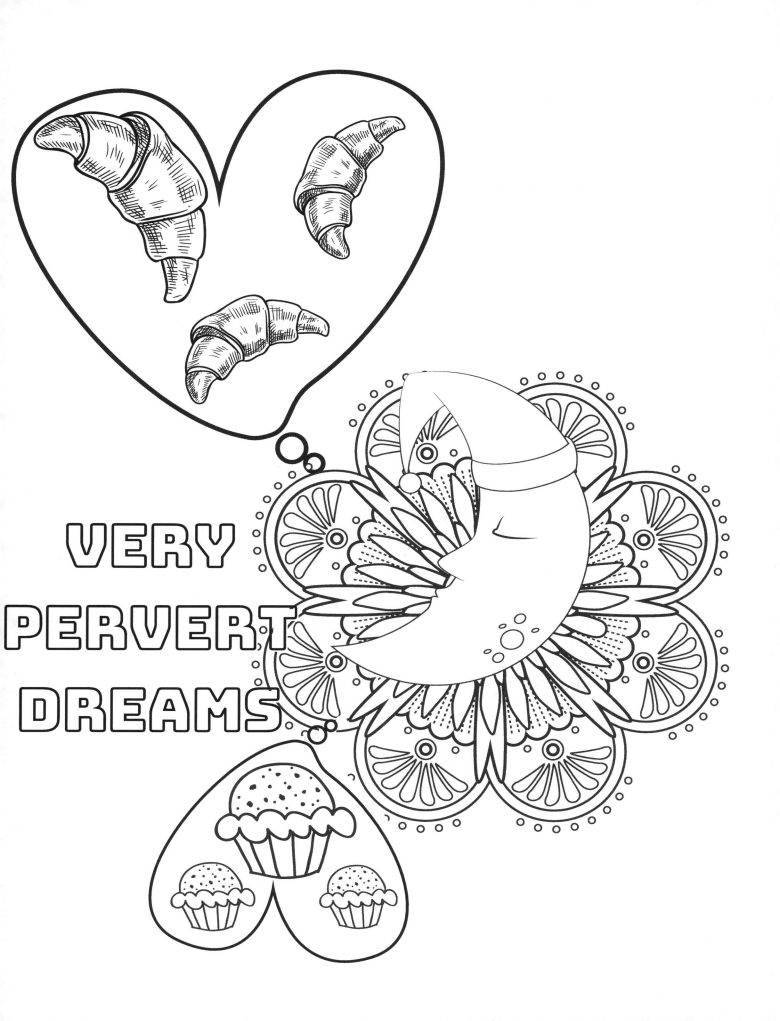

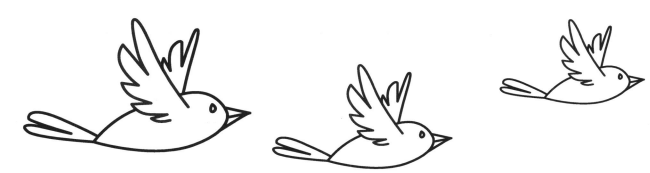

I'LL EAT MUSHROOMS ALL MY LIFE
THEY'RE GLUTEN-FREE, FOR SURE

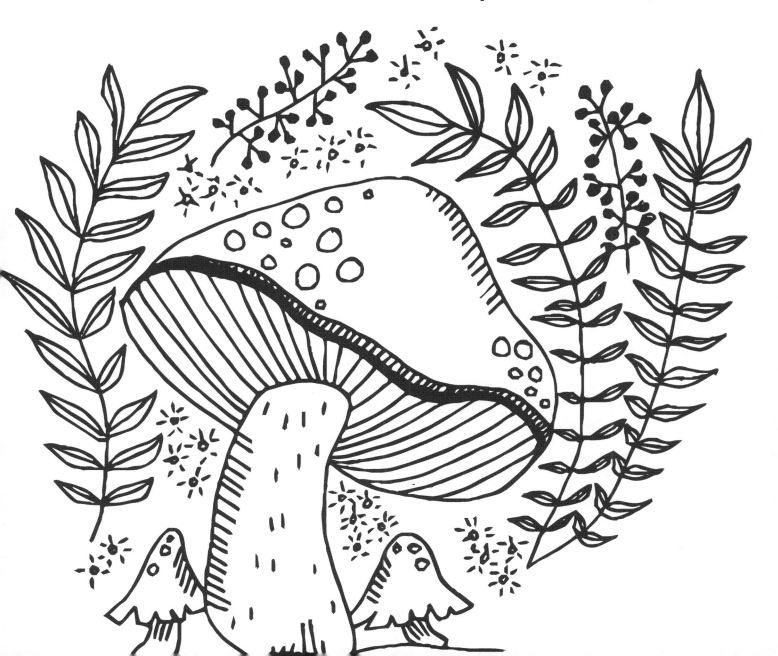

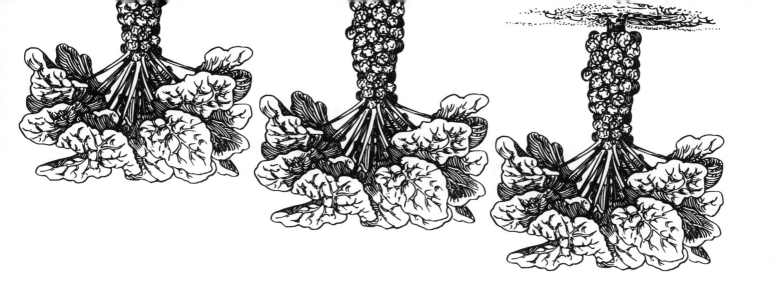

SOME RANDOM PLANT

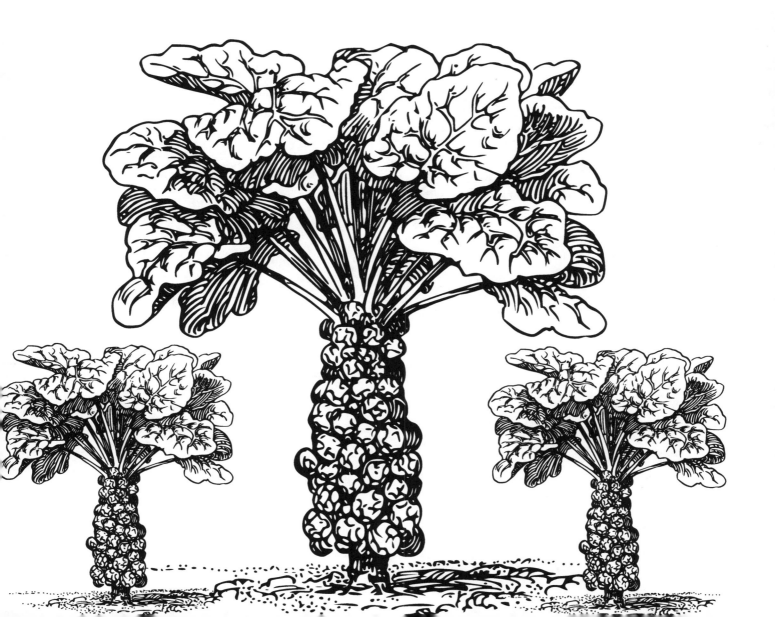

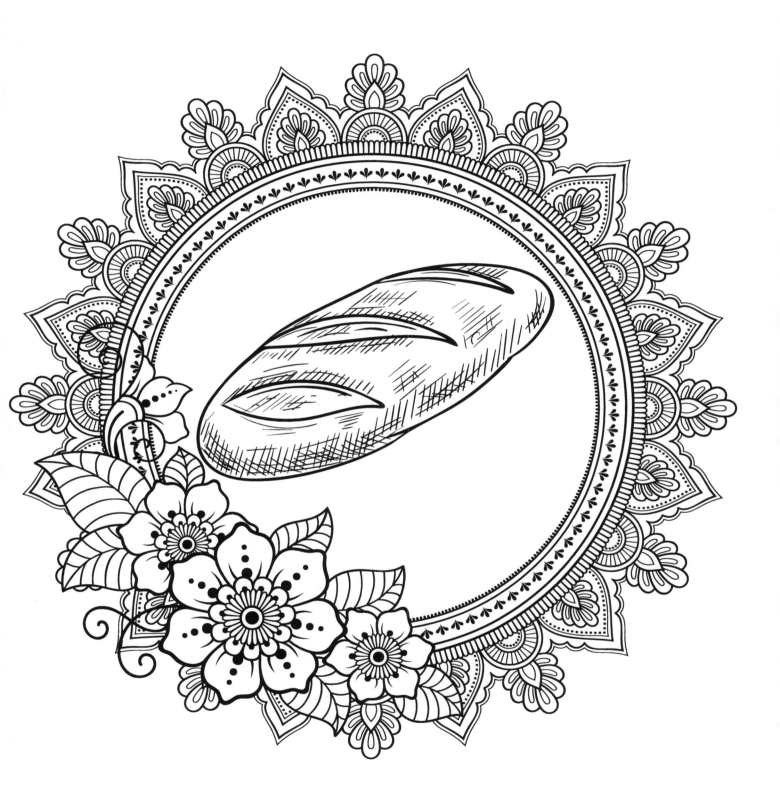

U CAN'T TOUCH THIS

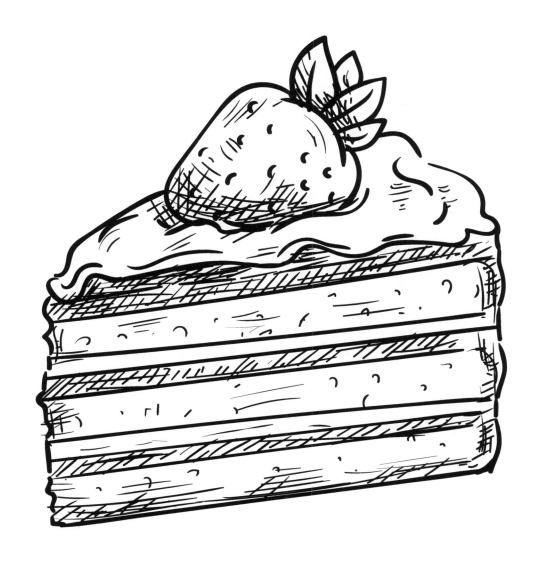

INGREDIENTS:
- YOU CAN'T EAT IT
- FORBIDDEN
- FUCK MY GENES

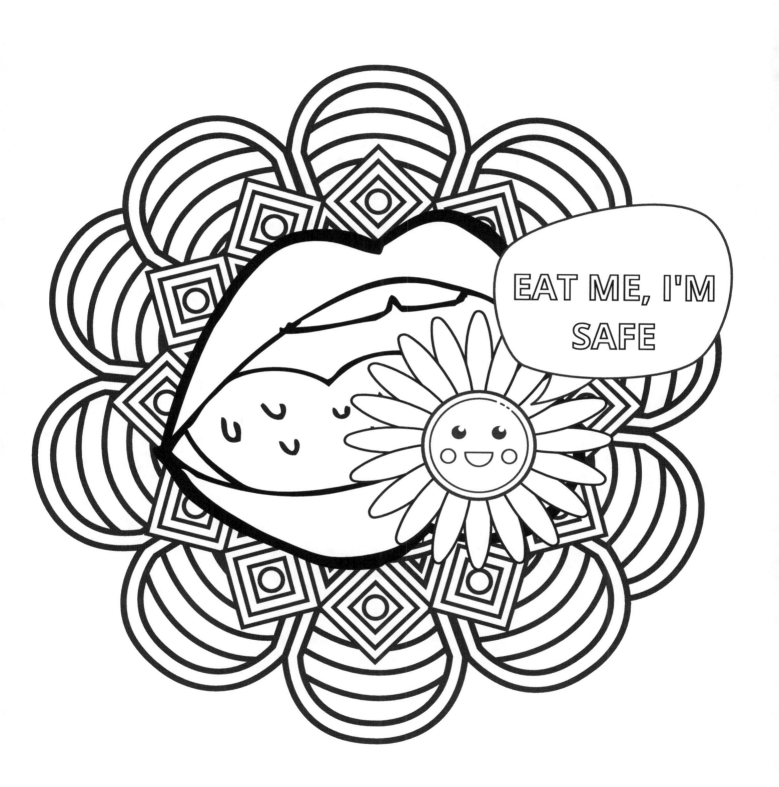

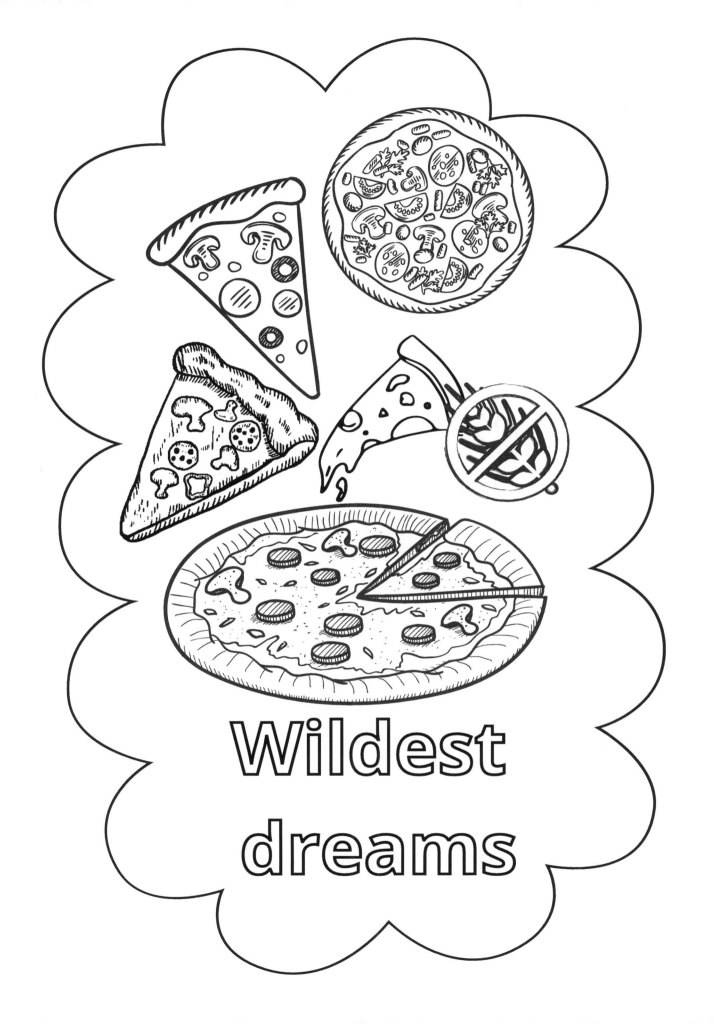

Wildest
dreams

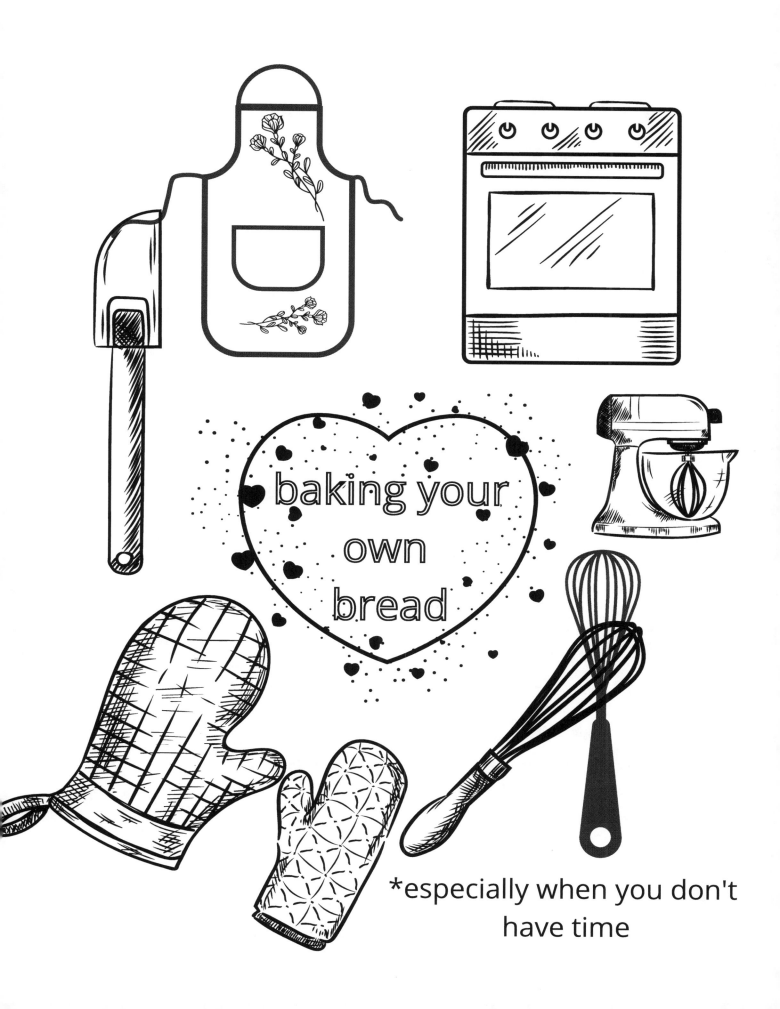

baking your
own
bread

*especially when you don't
have time

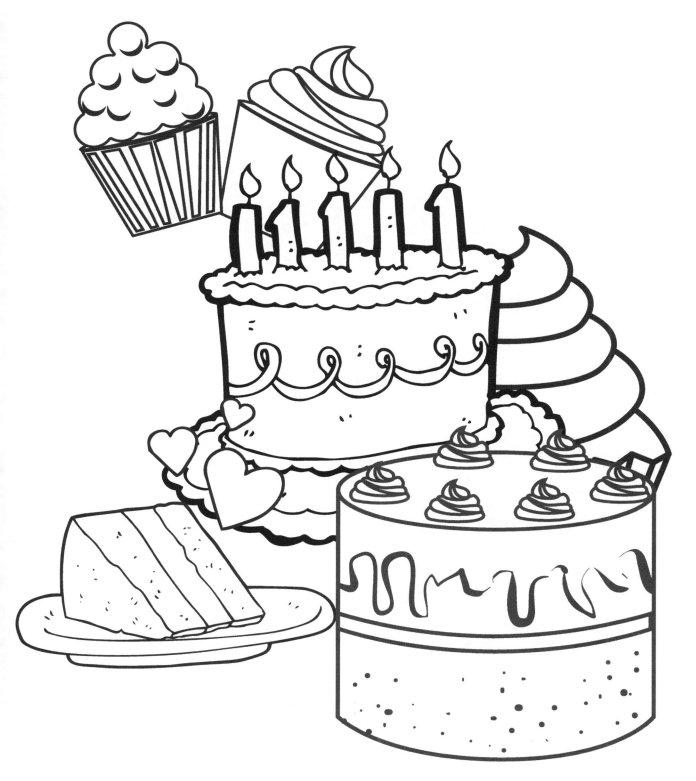

Make a wish...
I wish that my illness
magically goes away

WE LOOK INNOCENT BUT WE CAN EASILY KILL YOU

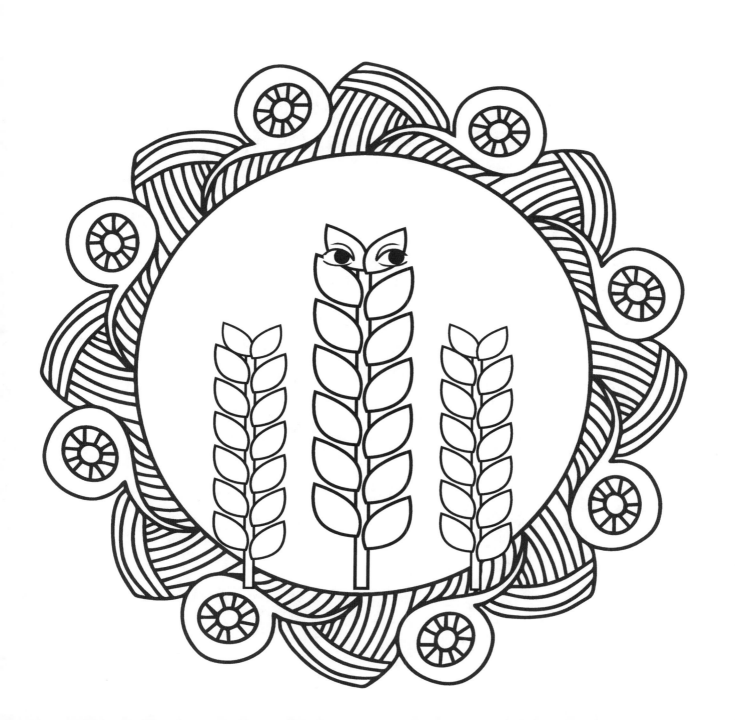

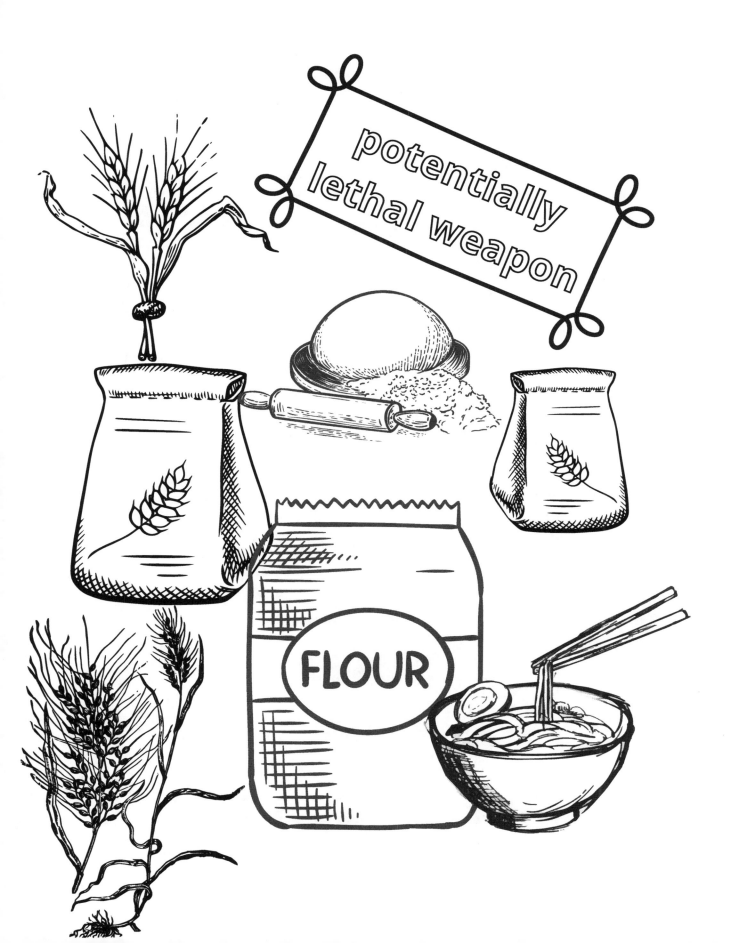

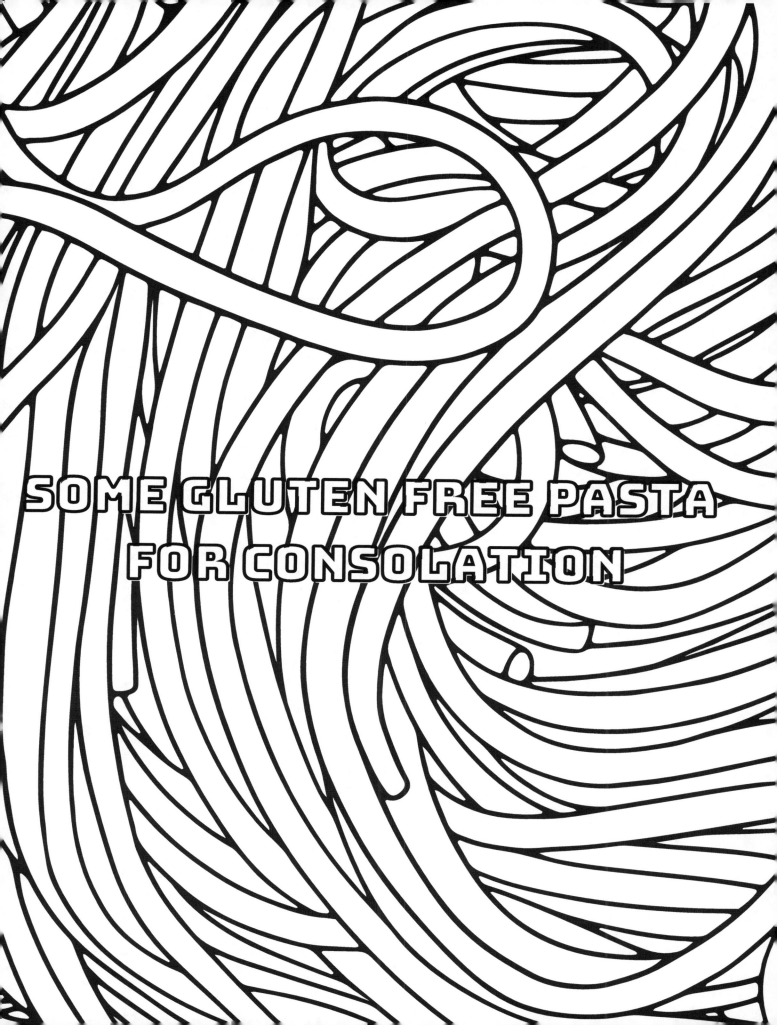

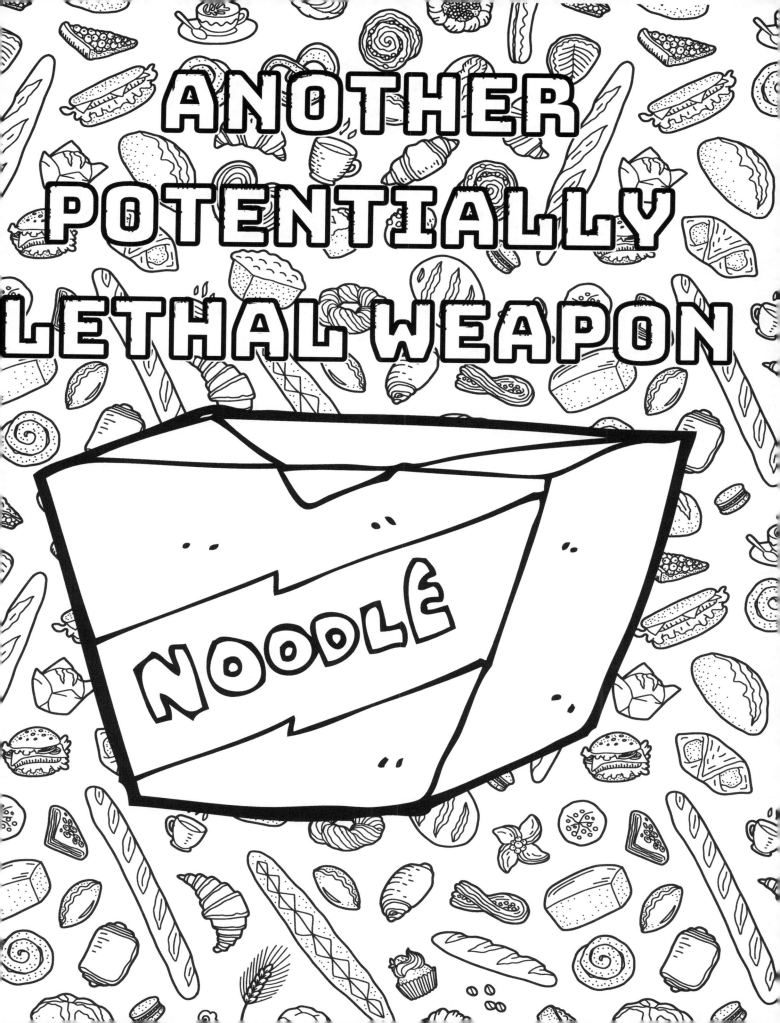

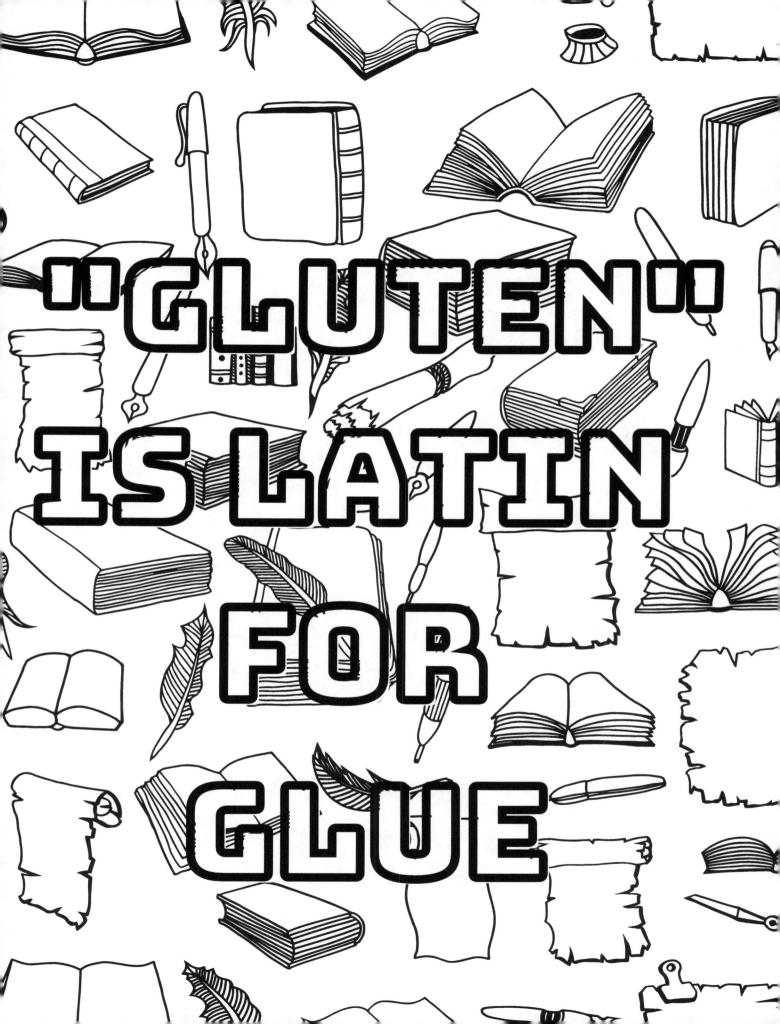

"GLUTEN" IS LATIN FOR GLUE

Hidden sources of gluten include licorice, alcohol, instant coffee, spices, soy sauce, and chewing gum.

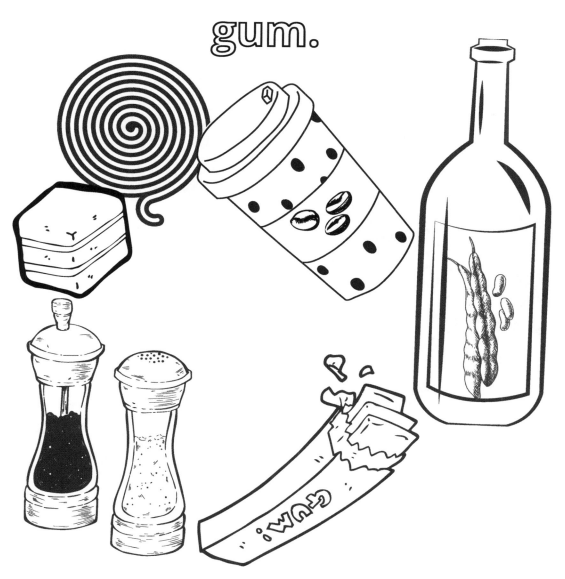

As if not eating 3/4 of all food wasn't hard enough

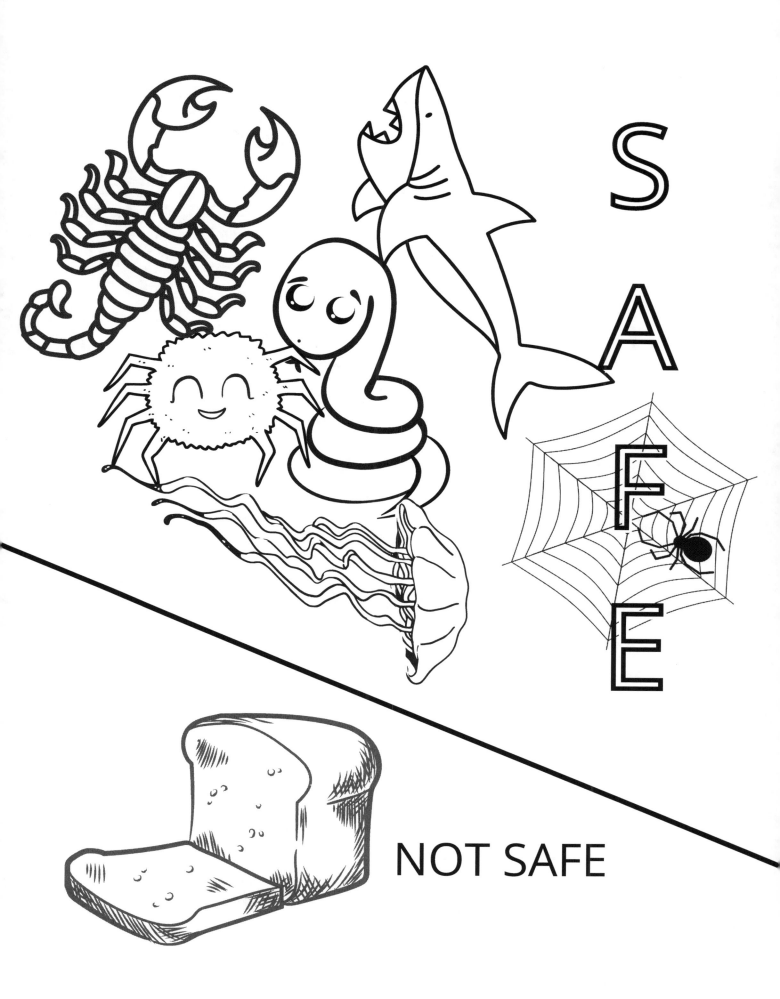

S
A
F
E

NOT SAFE

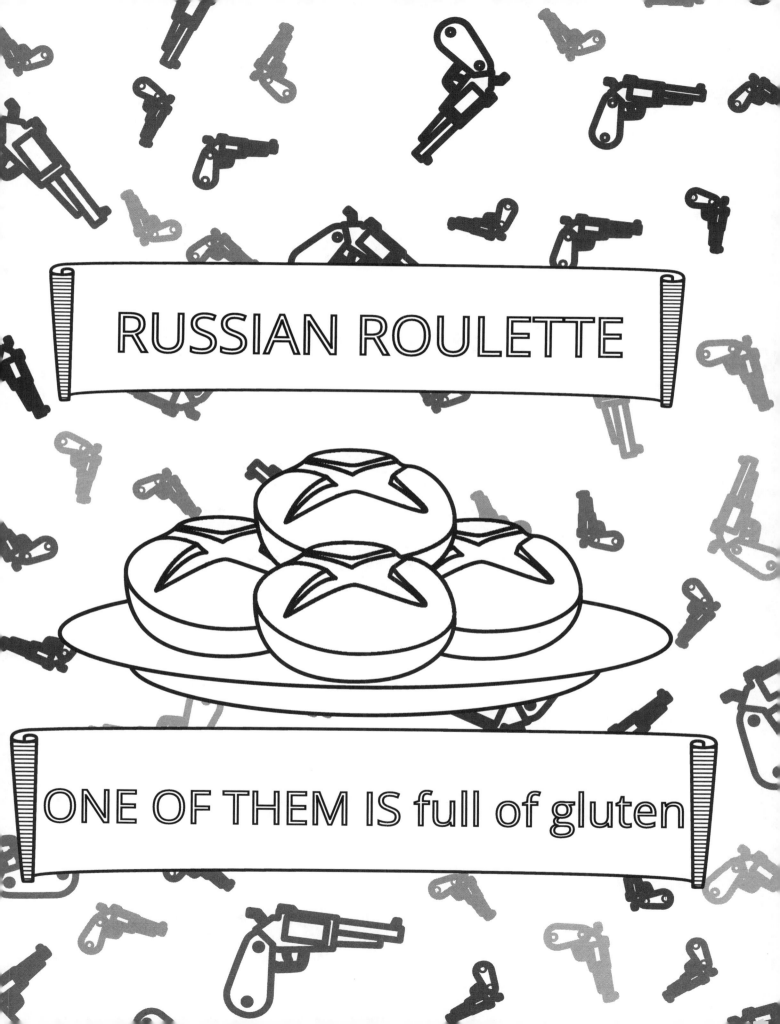

JAR OF GLUTEN-FREE TEARS

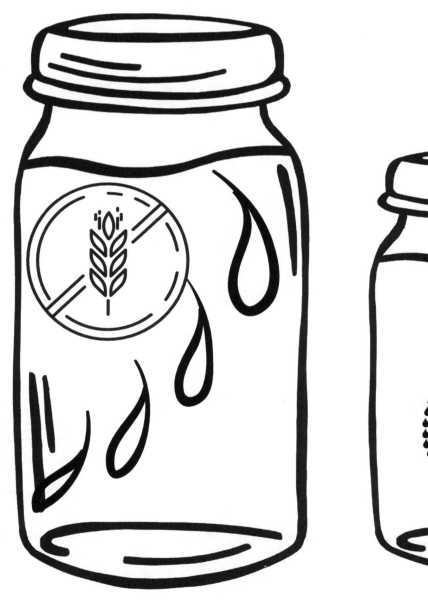
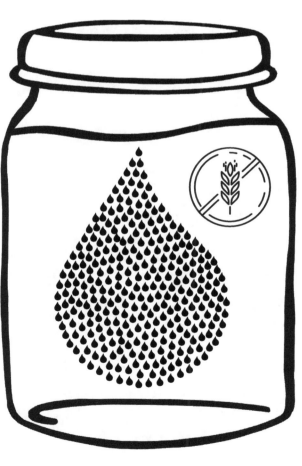

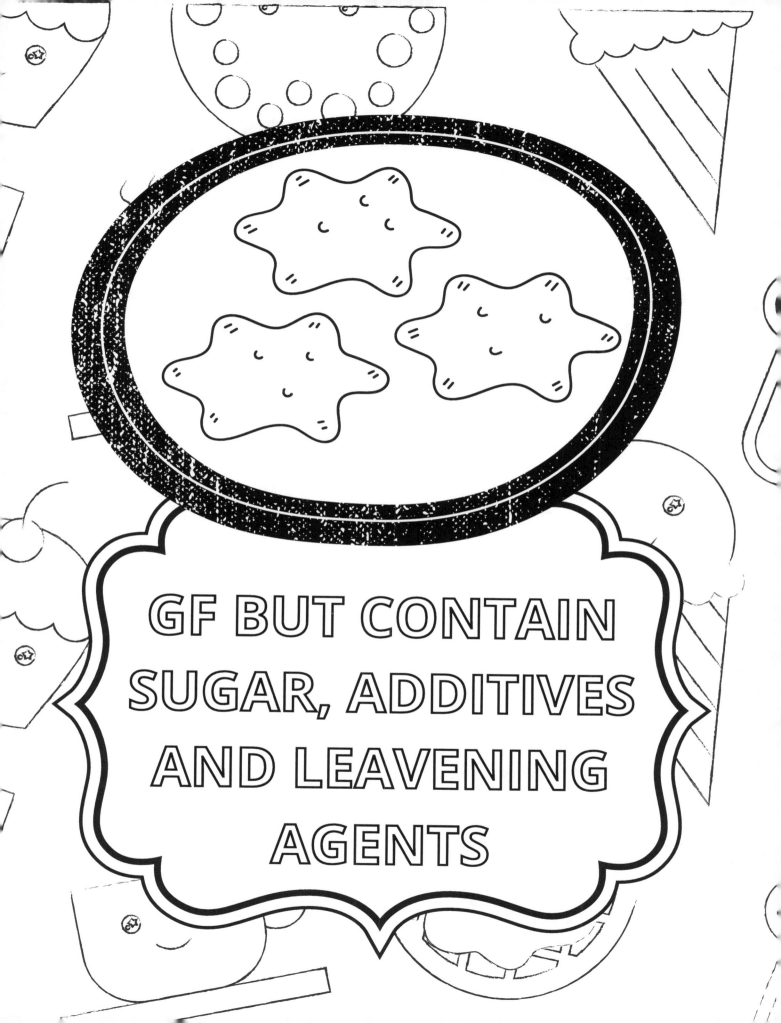

GF BUT CONTAIN SUGAR, ADDITIVES AND LEAVENING AGENTS

Maybe
gluten-free

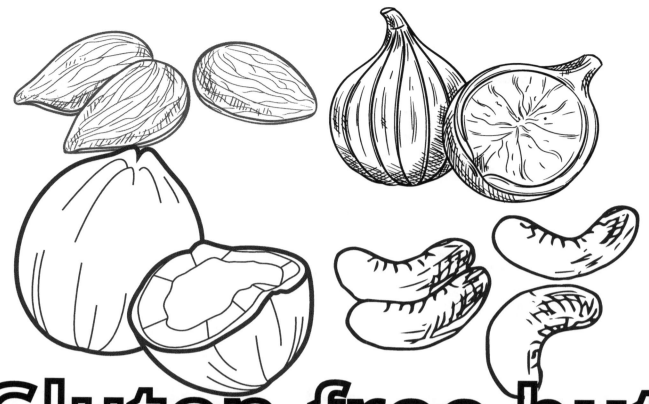

Gluten-free but trigger allergies

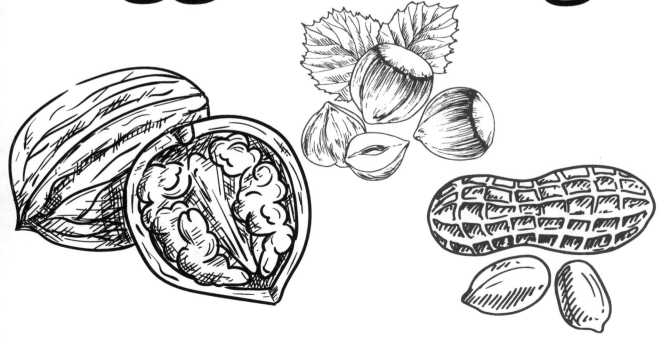

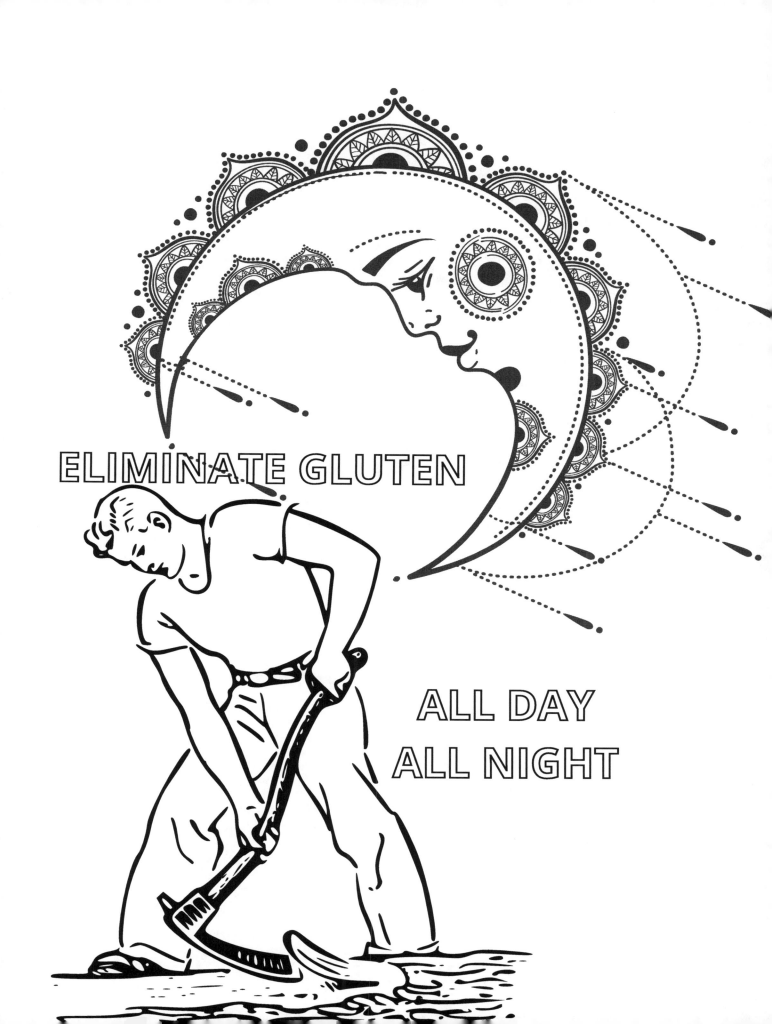

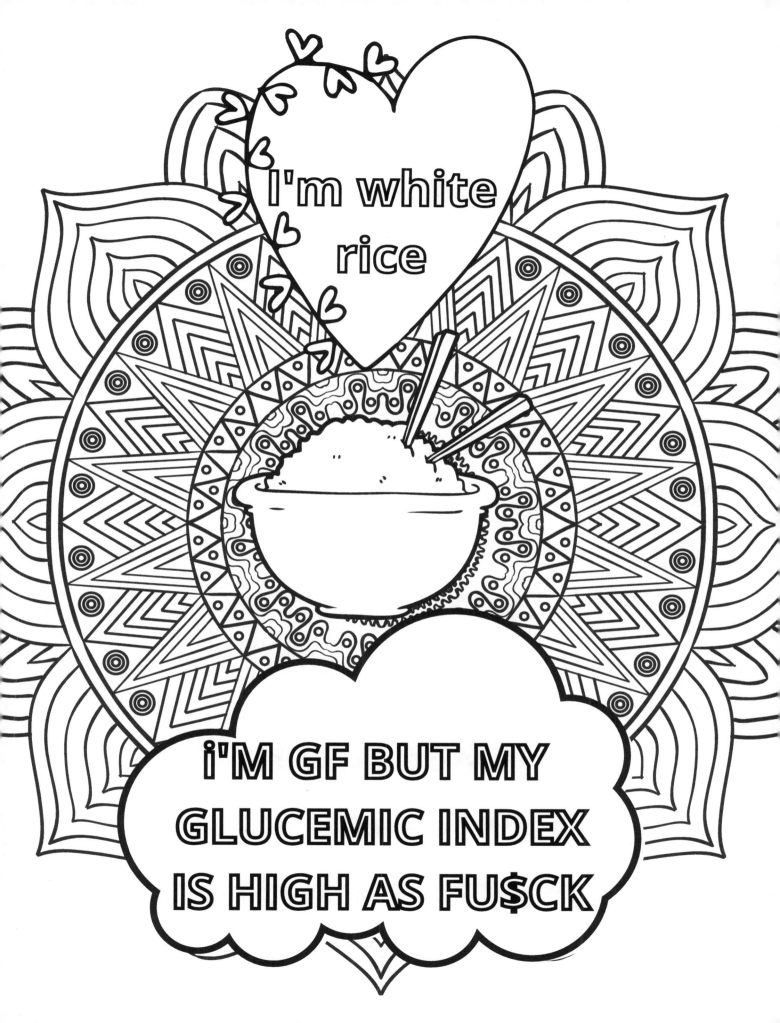

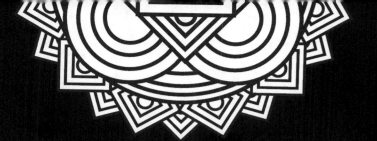

BREATHARIANISM

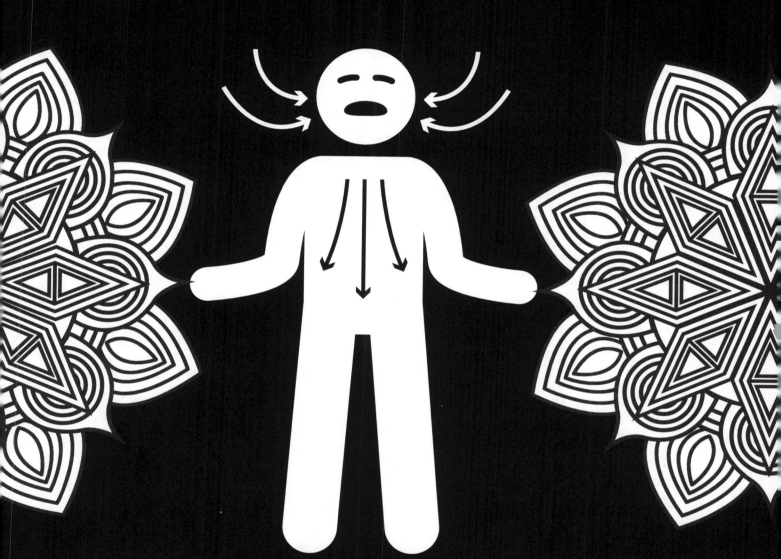

PERHAPS THE ONLY WAY
TO EAT GLUTEN-FREE

I'm fine!

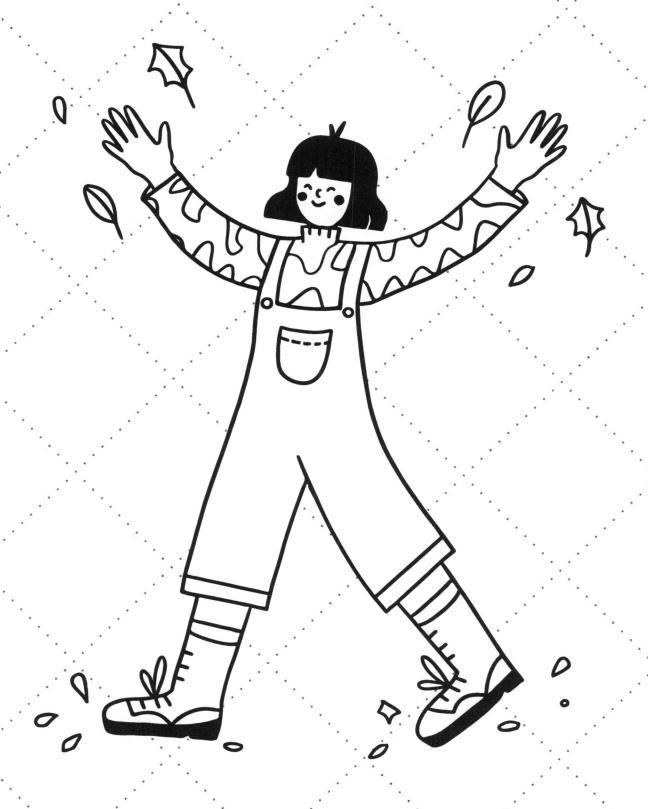

Made in the USA
Middletown, DE
26 June 2025

77537860R00038